Nadia Fettal
Nadjet Siali

Current status of COPD in Sidi Bel Abbes

Nadia Fettal
Nadjet Siali

Current status of COPD in Sidi Bel Abbes

ScienciaScripts

Table of contents

LIST OF FIGURES AND TABLES

List of figures

PART 1: LITERATURE REVIEW

I- INTRODUCTION

Chronic obstructive pulmonary disease (COPD) is a progressively progressive chronic inflammatory disease of the bronchi, mainly related to smoking, characterized by non-fully reversible bronchial obstruction of airflow[1].

COPD is a highly prevalent pathology, and its incidence is set to increase in the future as the population ages and smoking prevalence rises worldwide [2]. According to Fuhmar [3], its prevalence is 7.5%, with a tendency to stabilize in men and increase in women.

COPD is a real public health problem, and its impact is growing all the time: it is currently the 5th leading cause of death worldwide, and it is estimated that by 2020 it will be the 3^e leading cause of death worldwide, compared with 6^e in 1990 [2]. It is the leading respiratory cause of direct healthcare costs, with less than a quarter of patients (the most severe) generating more than half the expenditure, mainly through hospitalization.

It's an under-diagnosed disease, and one that's often overlooked by doctors [4]. The first bronchial symptoms (chronic cough and sputum) are trivialized, and culturally integrated with smoking: smokers therefore do not refer to them as the first manifestations of a real disease. Dyspnea, a frequent reason for consultation but a late symptom, reflects the onset of obstructive respiratory insufficiency.

COPD is incapacitating due to the progressive decline in respiratory function (FEV1): when FEV1 falls to 50%, dyspnea becomes incapacitating and the risk of respiratory failure becomes real, this is the stage of respiratory handicap. Below 30%, there is a risk of death from COPD [5].

It is a systemic pathology with respiratory origins. The evolution of COPD is complicated by extra-respiratory manifestations (cardiovascular, diabetes, osteoporosis, bronchial cancer, anemia, undernutrition....), engendered by the existence of low-grade systemic inflammation and the presence of common risk factors such as smoking, aging and a sedentary lifestyle. The occurrence of co-morbidities worsens the prognosis of the disease and contributes to the deterioration in quality of life of COPD patients [6,7].

The quality of life of COPD sufferers is severely impaired, even in the early stages of the disease [8,9,10], and learned societies are recommending the assessment of quality of life as a new parameter to be integrated alongside functional parameters in the overall management of COPD patients.

1-Definition of COPD

Several definitions of COPD have been drawn up by different learned societies (ATS, ERS), and have followed one another over time as knowledge of the disease has improved.

Definition (ATS 1995)[11]: permanent bronchial obstruction (documented by FEV1/CV<70%) due to chronic bronchitis or emphysema, or their combination. Bronchial obstruction is generally progressive, may be accompanied by bronchial hyperreactivity and may be partially reversible. Bronchial asthma is no longer included in COPD, nor are conditions of specific etiology such as cystic fibrosis or bronchiolitis obliterans.

Definition (GOLD 2002) [12]: COPD is a condition characterized by airflow limitation that is not completely reversible. Airflow limitation is progressive and most often associated with an abnormal inflammatory response of the lungs to noxious particulate or gaseous agents.

Definition (GOLD2006) [13]: COPD is a preventable and treatable disease. It has extrapulmonary manifestations that may contribute to its severity in some patients. The pulmonary component is characterized by airflow limitation, which is not reversible. Airflow limitation is usually progressive and associated with an abnormal inflammatory response of the lungs to noxious particulate or gaseous agents.

Definition (GOLD 2016) [14]: it is a preventable and treatable disease characterized by persistent expiratory flow limitation that is progressive and associated with an increased chronic inflammatory response in the airways and lung secondary to exposure to noxious particles or gases.

Exacerbations and comorbidities contribute to overall severity in sick individuals.

The term COPD has replaced the former terms chronic bronchitis and emphysema. However, COPD is not synonymous with chronic bronchitis and emphysema. In simpler terms, it includes chronic bronchitis, emphysema or a combination of the two. It also includes patients without signs of chronic bronchitis or radiological evidence of pulmonary emphysema.

The definition of chronic bronchitis is clinical; chronic cough and sputum for at least 3 months a year and for at least two consecutive years, with no other cause identified [15].the presence of chronic bronchitis should prompt a search for COPD by spirometry.the diagnosis is retained if the FEV1/CV<70% ratio after administration of a bronchodilator. The absence of bronchitis does not exclude COPD. The rate of patients presenting with COPD without cough or sputum varies according to the series, from 26 to 90% of cases, and seems to decrease with the severity of COPD [16 ,17].

Emphysema is defined anatomically as abnormal and permanent enlargement of the airspace beyond the terminal bronchioles, associated with destruction of the alveolar walls. A distinction is made between centrilobular emphysema, which affects the central region of the acinus and is an integral part of the peripheral anatomical lesions of COPD, and pan-lobular emphysema, characterized by destruction of all acinus components. It is often associated with the most severe forms of α 1-antitrypsin deficiency [18].

2-   Determinants of lung function decline

2.1/Bronchial hyperreactivity: This may play a role in the decline of respiratory function. The lung health study[19] showed that in non-asthmatic smokers aged 35-59 with an FEV1/CV<70% ratio, the level of bronchial reactivity to methacholine was the second most important predictor of FEV1 decline, after smoking. This bronchial hyperactivity was greater in active smokers than in ex-smokers.

2.2/-Genetic factors: Apart from the genetic deficiency of a-1antitrypsin, which is responsible for the onset of early and severe emphysema, there are other genetic factors [20]. There is a genetic predisposition that may explain the onset and development of COPD in certain "susceptible" smokers.This involves a genetic imbalance in other well-defined systems: protease-antiproteinase balance (alpha-1-ati-chymotrypsin, alpha-2macroglobulin, matrix metalloproteinases, antioxidant enzymes (heme oxygenase-1), inflammatory mediators (vitamin D carrier protein, TNF-alpha, IL-1 complex), factors involved in mucociliary clearance (CFTR).In certain patients with a particular genetic make-up, it would seem that inhalation of toxic smoke could modulate the host's response by acting on the decline in FEV1.

2.3/Smoking toxicity: Smoking is recognized as a key factor in the development of COPD. Persistent smoking exacerbates the decline in FEV1, as demonstrated by Fletcher and Peto[21]. Conversely, in weaned smokers, FEV1 improves, in line with the natural evolution of lung function (Figure 1).

Figure 1: The Fletcher curve of FEV1 decline in relation to smoking

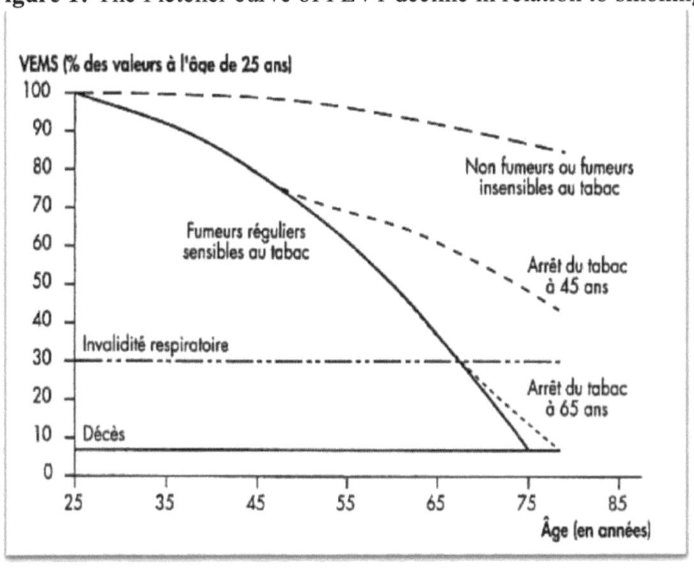

2.4/Exacerbations: Exacerbations accelerate the progression of COPD, by further reducing FEV1. This inflammation is heightened during exacerbations of infectious origin, responsible for bronchospasm and mucosal edema. Repeated episodes worsen bronchial obstruction, further limiting airflow [21,22].

Donalson's team [22] showed that COPD subjects with more than three exacerbations per year experienced a more rapid decline in FEV1 than other COPD subjects over a four-year follow-up period: -4.22% versus -3.59%.

Another North American study [23] was a multicenter study of 5887 smokers aged 35-60 years, with the aim of monitoring the decline in FEV1 by EFR follow-up over 5 years. This study revealed that a single lower respiratory infection caused an additional decline in FEV1 of 7ml/year. Persistent smoking associated with frequent lower respiratory infections (more than 1.5

episodes) resulted in a greater decline in FEV1, averaging 69.4ml versus 13.1ml/year in weaned patients with fewer than 0.24 exacerbations/year.

2.5/The role of drugs

With the exception of the TORCH study, all the long-term studies (LHS, CCHS, EUROSCOP, ISOLDE, BRONCUS, UPLIFT) used FEV1 decline as the primary endpoint, and a treatment that slows FEV1 decline is considered to influence the natural course of the disease. Among the drugs enrolled in clinical trials: corticoids, tiotropium, ipratropium bromide and N-acetylcysteine.

No study using FEV1 decline as an efficacy criterion has demonstrated any effect of treatment on this functional parameter.

3-   Exacerbations

3-1Definition: These are acute episodes of disease aggravation occurring during the course of the disease. They affect all stages of COPD severity, with variable frequency. They have a negative impact on lung function and quality of life, and increase mortality rates and healthcare costs.

There is no universal definition, despite several attempts at consensus [24], and definitions vary according to the recommendations of learned societies or the criteria taken into account. Consensus defines an exacerbation as an exacerbation of pre-existing dyspnea, associated with cough and/or sputum in a COPD patient requiring therapeutic modification (GOLD 2006).

A recent study by Jones et al [25] developed a more quantitative definition of COPD exacerbations, based on 14 items selected from a list of 150, resulting in a score called EEXACT-PRO.

3.2- Frequency of exacerbations

Exacerbations can occur at any stage of COPD, with an average frequency of 2 to 3 episodes per year [26,27], depending on the patient. This figure is high considering the major impact on the patient and his or her disease. It is probably underestimated, as shown by the study by Seemungal et al. in which 50% of exacerbations defined as a worsening of symptoms were not reported by patients [20]. However, most of these corresponded to exacerbations classified as mild, with criteria such as the common cold.

Some patients with frequent exacerbations have a particularly high number of exacerbations [27].

The frequency and severity of exacerbations increase with the severity of COPD [28,29,30].

3.3- Healthcare costs

Exacerbations lead to increased use of healthcare resources (hospitalizations, urgent medical visits, treatment consumption, home care) and are responsible for 60% of the direct costs of COPD[30] themselves estimated at between 3 and 9 billion euros per year and 3-9% of healthcare expenditure in France[31].

Exacerbations put a strain on the budget of social organizations, mainly due to hospitalization costs. Hospitalization accounts for 40-57% of COPD-related healthcare costs, rising to 63% for severe patients [32]. In Spain, the average cost of an exacerbation of any severity is €193, while in Sweden, mild exacerbations managed by the patient cost €13, while those requiring hospitalization average €2,300 [33].

3.4- Physiological consequences of exacerbations

The exacerbation is linked to an increase in pre-existing airway inflammation associated with a rise in the colonizing bacterial load or the acquisition of a new bacterial species. The presence of a bacterial infection favors the release of proinflammatory cytokines, a local influx of neutrophils and increased secretion of proteinases. These pathophysiological changes give rise to bronchospasm, which is responsible for dyspnea, and bronchial hypersecretion, leading to coughing and expectoration. However, the inflammatory process differs from one exacerbation to another and depends on the etiology [19].

In non-bacterial exacerbations, exacerbations secondary to pathogenic bacteria are characterized by inflammation rich in neutrophils, IL-8, tumor necrosis factor (TNF) alpha and leukocyte elastase [19].

3.5- Impact of exacerbations on the COPD patient

The negative impact of exacerbations felt by patients relates to their daily life, the need to seek care, increased dyspnoea and coughing, sleep disturbance, fear of recurrence, hospitalization and confinement to home or bed, anxiety and psychological distress. The patients of Haughney et al [34] confirmed that impairment of daily life was the main impact of exacerbations.

3.5.1- Impact on respiratory function

*Short-term: variations in expiratory flow rate (PEF), FEV1 and forced vital capacity (FVC) are generally small in amplitude, but are greater during severe exacerbations. PEF falls by a median of 8.6l/min, FEV1 by 24ml and forced vital capacity by 76ml [19]. A cohort study involving 101 COPD patients assessed FEV1 and PEF before, during and after an exacerbation[20], revealing little change in either functional parameter compared with dyspnoea, which worsens in 70% of cases. Time to recovery of initial PEF values is longer>35 days in 25% of patients.

Dynamic distension is aggravated by exacerbations, as demonstrated by Parker et al[35], and is associated with a change in reactance and limitation of respiratory flow[36,37].

Severe exacerbations alter gas exchange by increasing ventilation-perfusion inequalities[38].

*Donalson et al [22] showed that the FEV1 of patients with three or more exacerbations per year declined faster than that of other patients: -4.22% versus -3.59%.

Recurrent exacerbations have a negative impact on the natural history of the disease, contributing to a worsening of the rate of decline in lung function.Thus ,the London team analyzed the slope of FEV1 decline over time over 4 years as a function of the frequency of exacerbations observed in their cohort.Patients with frequent exacerbations the rate of decline in FEV1 was 8ml/year greater than those with fewer exacerbations [23].

3.5.2- Impact on COPD composite scores

The authors [39] observed a lasting deterioration in the BODE score secondary to changes in respiratory function, muscle strength and physical activity during COPD exacerbations. The score increased (+1.1 points at 2 years) without returning to baseline in patients who had experienced at least one exacerbation, whereas it remained unchanged in patients without exacerbations [40].All components of the score were affected, but it was the walking test that decreased significantly compared with baseline [41].

3.5.3- Impact on cardiovascular risk

The risk of cardiovascular disease is elevated during exacerbations; an increased incidence of myocardial infarction is observed within five days, and stroke within seven weeks of exacerbation [42,43].exacerbations increase vascular risk, probably through common mechanisms related to infection and acute inflammation, and the risk of pulmonary embolism [44,45].

The negative effect of exacerbation treatments may contribute to cardiovascular risk The use of oral corticosteroids is thought to increase the risk of MI [46], while high-dose β2-agonist bronchodilators may have adverse cardiac effects [47].Conversely, β-blockers appear to exert a protective effect on mortality [48].

Elevations in cardiac troponin and NT-proBNP are strong evidence of myocardial injury induced by COPD exacerbations [49].

3.5.4- Impact on quality of life

Exacerbations have a negative short- and medium-term impact on all areas of quality of life, as shown by a study by the team of Bourbeau et al [50], who demonstrated that all dimensions of quality of life are impaired from the start of the exacerbation and during the 15 days that follow, compared with the baseline state (excluding the exacerbation). Recovery of mental health status takes 39 days, compared with 18 days for daily activity.

Deterioration in quality of life increases with the number of exacerbations (three or more)[52].

A recent study showed that 30% of relatives showed some signs of post-traumatic stress disorder, revealed within 90 days of admission [53].

3.5.5- Impact on mortality

Mortality rates in patients hospitalized for COPD exacerbations vary from 5 to 60%, depending on the severity of the disease[19].

Exacerbations are a significant cause of death, particularly in stage III and IV COPD, accounting for 43 per 1000 individuals, i.e. eight times more deaths than in the general population [19].

Mortality in COPD patients increases after a hospitalized exacerbation, with a critical period of 4.4 months after exacerbations when mortality is around 15%, and a mortality rate of 40-50% two years after hospitalization for a COPD exacerbation[54].

Exacerbations requiring intensive care are associated with a mortality of 24% to 30%[55].Risk factors for mortality in COPD exacerbations are age, comorbidity score, FEV1, body mass index (BMI) and long-term home oxygen therapy (LTO).Mortality is also correlated with the frequency of severe exacerbations, independent of the preceding factors[56].

3.6-Clinical signs and severity of exacerbations

Symptoms considered in the identification of COPD are cough, sputum and dyspnoea, and some studies consider systemic criteria (Table 1) such as fever [53].

Table 1: Clinical descriptors used to characterize acute COPD exacerbations, adapted from Anthonisen and Rodriguez-Roisin[53].

Category	Descriptor
Respiratory	Increased breathlessness Increased sputum volume and purulence Increased coughing Shallow/fast breathing
Systemic	Temperature rise Increased heart rate Altered mental state

3.6.1-Assessing signs of severity

The prognosis of an exacerbation depends on several criteria, such as in-hospital mortality, the need for assisted ventilation, admission to intensive care, length of hospital stay and last exacerbation recurrence [54].

Certain features of the patient and of the pathology can predict in-hospital mortality: high age, male sex, persistent smoking, presence of comorbidities, frequent hospital admissions, rest dyspnea, severe basic bronchial obstruction, undernutrition, and impaired gas exchange requiring long-term oxygen therapy[55].

3.6.2-Clinical examination data

The clinical criteria for exacerbation severity are intensity of dyspnoea, increase in RF, HR, signs of hypercapnia, alertness disorders, muscle fatigue and use of accessory respiratory muscles, and gasometric disorders, hypoalbunemia and elevated CRP[56].Table 2 summarizes the signs of exacerbation severity.

3.7-Etiologies of exacerbations

A/-Tracheobronchial infections

The etiologies of hospitalized COPD exacerbations are most often infectious (table 3); bacterial in 30%, viral in 25% and bacterial and viral in 25%. In the literature, bacterial or viral etiology is found in 70-80% of exacerbations requiring hospitalization[19].

Table 2;Initial signs of severity of COPD exacerbations

Patient history
High age
Socioeconomic precarious
Hospitalization in the last 06 months
Multiple hospitalizations during the current year
Severe rest dyspnea
Severe limitation of activities, bedridden subject

FEV1<35% of theoretical value
Rapid and significant deterioration in respiratory function
Existence of pulmonary hypertension
Long-term oxygen therapy
Corticosteroid therapy
Comorbidities
Undernutrition
Clinical examination data
Importance of dyspnea
Cyanosis
Confusion, coma, asterixis
Lower limb oedemas
Use of accessory respiratory muscles

Certain prodromal symptoms, such as nasal obstruction and rhinorrhea, are suggestive of viral exacerbations, in addition to the presence of seroconversion to several viruses. In 60% of cases, exacerbations are due to rhinovirus, influenza virus or respiratory syncytial virus [57], identified by polymerase chain reaction (PCR) from nasopharyngeal secretions of exacerbated patients. Viral infection may precede bacterial infection. Certain viruses can predispose to specific bacterial infections: influenza virus, streptococcus pneumonae or staphylococcus aureus during pneumonia and possibly during exacerbations[58].

Table 3: The list of germs responsible for exacerbations of COPD[19]

Bacteria	Virus
Haemophilus influenzae	Rhinovirus
Streptococcus pneumoniae	Influenza

Moraxella catarrhalis	Para-influenza
Haemophilus para-influenzae	Coronavirus
Staphylococcus aureus	Adenovirus
Pseudomonas aerugenosa spp.	Respiratory syncytial virus
Stenotrophomonas spp	Picornavirus
Other gram-negative bacilli	Metapneumovirus

Regarding bacterial etiology, the etiological mechanism of an exacerbation is the increase in the bacterial load naturally present in the stable airways of COPD patients[19]. During exacerbations, the proportion of pathogenic bacteria found in the airways is 25% with sputum cytobacteriological tests (ECB) and 61% with bronchial aspirates.The acquisition of a new bacterial strain is associated with a doubling of the risk of exacerbation within 4 to 8 weeks[19].

The onset of an exacerbation is not necessarily associated with the acquisition of a new germ, but can also occur following quantitative and qualitative variations in the bacterial load of an already colonizing strain [19].

BZ-Other causes

The impaired mucociliary clearance observed in COPD patients makes them more susceptible to the pro-inflammatory effects of certain inhaled pollutants, which secondarily aggravate airway damage. Other causes include interruptions in background treatment or the use of certain medications (psychotropic drugs, diuretics), left-sided cardiac dysfunction, pulmonary embolism and pneumonia. In a third of cases, no cause is found [19].

4-Comorbidities

COPD is an inflammatory pathology with systemic tropism and a respiratory starting point[59].chronic pathologies, including COPD, rarely occur in isolation. COPD patients frequently suffer from other extrarespiratory diseases such as cardiovascular disease, hypertension, diabetes, osteoporosis and undernutrition....

Charlson et al [60] reported in a study of 5861 chronically ill subjects that 65% of COPD sufferers had one or two chronic pathologies (hypertension, diabetes, cardiovascular disease, depression, osteoporosis, cancer, etc.).

The frequency of comorbidities was found in another EABPCO study[60], carried out on COPD patients hospitalized for an exacerbation (table 4).

The links between COPD and other chronic extra-respiratory pathologies are represented by the risk factors of aging, tobacco intoxication and genetic predisposition. However, there is a direct link for certain comorbidities, notably cardiovascular disease, metabolic disease and cancer, and this would be the presence of low-grade systemic inflammation in this population [61,62].

Since 2006 [63], the definition of COPD has been revised to include the association of extra-respiratory manifestations.

Table 4: The frequency of comorbidities in COPD

Age (years)	M± AND	70.3± 11.3
Age	<60 years	19.9
	60-79 years	56.9
	≥80 years	23.2
BMI	≤20kg/m2	20.3
	20-25kg/m2	34.5
	25-30kg/m2	26.7
Right-hand heart %.	Secondary PAH	7.4
	Chronic IVD	4.6
Comorbidities, %.	Heart disease ischemic	19.0
		12.7
	Heart failure	35.1

	HTA	7.3
	Sleep apnea syndrome	2.5
	Cancers	

These comorbidities associated with COPD can worsen the patient's vital prognosis, as was clearly detailed in the analysis of causes of death in the TORCH study[65].It is well established that the accumulation of comorbidities is associated with excess mortality [66] and increased healthcare costs[60].

Corlateanu et al [67] assessed quality of life using the Saint George Questionnaire (SGDJ) in two groups of COPD patients: those under 65 and those over 65. This study revealed that the number of comorbidities correlated with impaired quality of life in elderly patients, but not in young COPD patients.

Comorbidities are an essential part of COPD management, due to their high frequency and negative impact on patients' quality of life and vital prognosis.

Although the level of bronchial obstruction was long considered to be the only parameter indicative of the severity and progression of the disease, we now know that there are other parameters of severity, including the presence of chronic diseases associated with COPD. Indeed, Burgel et al have proposed a new classification of COPD severity with four phenotypes [68].

4.1-From pulmonary to systemic inflammation

Previous studies have demonstrated an increase in plasma concentrations of inflammatory markers (TNF-α)[69] and other non-specific mediators, such as acute-phase proteins (IL-6, etc.). Moreover, the severity of this systemic inflammation increases with time and during COPD exacerbations[69].

A causal relationship between the sites of inflammation can therefore be envisaged in both directions: either the respiratory manifestations of COPD result from the pulmonary localization of a systemic inflammation, or the systemic inflammation is the consequence of a dissemination of the pulmonary inflammation of COPD.

The correlation between the severity of one and the other [70] is not conclusive, but the presence of specific markers of pulmonary inflammation in the circulation, such as surfactant protein D [70], argues in favor of the second hypothesis.

Among the cytokines of systemic inflammation, IL-6, which contributes to increased acute-phase protein concentration, TNF-a, IL- 1β, chemokineCXCL8 (IL-8) and adipokines (leptins and ghrelin) play a potential role in comorbidities.Increased CRP, fibrinogen, serum amyloid apolipoprotein A or surfactant protein D are often related to the severity of exacerbations[71]

A/-Cardiovascular pathologies :

Cardiovascular pathologies are at the forefront (35% hypertension, 19% left heart failure, 13% ischemic heart disease). This frequency is explained by the presence of risk factors common to both pathologies (smoking, ageing, genetic factors).

However, SIN et al. have shown that a fall in FEV1 is a mortality risk factor independent of age, sex and smoking [62].

In patients with mild-to-moderate COPD, the authors found that a 10% reduction in predicted FEV1 was associated with a 28% increase in the frequency of fatal coronary events.

Almost half of all cases die of cardiovascular events. The risk of dying from a cardiovascular event is markedly increased in patients with COPD compared to a control population of the same age and sex without COPD.

The mechanisms involved in the pathogenesis of cardiovascular disease in COPD patients are diverse: the systemic inflammatory process, hypoxia, oxidative stress and activation of the sympathetic nervous system, as well as connective tissue remodeling processes. Together, these factors promote vascular dysfunction.

B/-Bronchial cancer

Bronchial cancer and COPD are two of the most frequent and deadly pathologies worldwide. These complications of smoking have interrelated and not totally independent mechanisms [73].

Depending on the study, the prevalence of bronchial cancer varies from 9-20% in COPD patients [72].

On the pathophysiological level, the authors evoke the theory of chronic inflammation of the airways with the accumulation of innate cells in the extracellular matrix; in fact, bronchial hypersecretion and the defect in mucociliary clearance of particles accentuate the concentration and duration of persistence of inhaled particles in certain zones of the bronchial tree[74].These effects may explain the increased risk of central bronchial cancer in COPD sufferers and the link between COPD severity and cancer risk[75].

Bronchial cancer is more common in COPD patients than in subjects with normal lung function. Numerous studies involving thousands of subjects, matched on smoking status, have shown that the presence of bronchial obstruction multiplies the risk of developing lung cancer by 2.23 in men and 3.97 in women, even in ex-smokers [76,77].

Impaired lung function, even for mild functional losses, and the presence of emphysema are two independent predictors of bronchial cancer [78].

Similarly, an accelerated decline in lung function associated with worsening disease would significantly increase the risk of lung cancer [75].

C/-Metabolic syndrome

The metabolic syndrome is characterized by a set of asymptomatic physiological and biochemical disturbances that may coexist with genetic and acquired factors. According to the WHO[79] ; it is the association of glucose intolerance, hyperinsulinemia or diabetes associated with at least two other metabolic abnormalities among :hypertension ^140/90mmhg or antihypertensive treatment, dyslipidemia(triglyceride level≥ 1.5g/l and/or HDL cholesterol< 0.35g/l for men and 0.39g/l for women),visceral or central obesity(waist/hip circumference ratio >0.9 for men and > 0.85 for women and/or
BMI>30kg/m2),others(urinary albumin excretion rate ≥ 20ug/min or albumin/creatinine ratio >30)mg/g).

COPD represents a significant risk factor (× 1.5-1.8) for the development of type 2 diabetes, even in moderately affected patients [79,66].

The prevalence of metabolic syndrome is reported to be 2 times higher in COPD patients than in age- and sex-matched healthy subjects[81], and a German study[82] suggests that it affects over 50% of COPD patients.

Reduced physical activity and inflammation via pro-inflammatory cytokines elevated in COPD, such as TNF alpha and interleukin 6, promote insulin resistance and potentiate the development of diabetes [83,84].

The presence of metabolic syndrome significantly increases the risk of developing diabetes, heart disease and stroke [85].

D/-Anemia

Anemia is often found in chronic respiratory pathologies, particularly COPD[86].Several studies have noted the high frequency of anemia in COPD patients[87,88].Its incidence is 10-30% depending on the study[89,90].It is generally a moderate anemia(HB<10g/dl) of the inflammatory, normochromic, normocytic and aregenerative type.

Anemia is associated with increased dyspnea, limited physical activity and high mortality[91,92].

Anemia is more frequent than polycythemia in COPD patients[93,94].

This anemia is related to systemic inflammation, functional martial deficiency, decreased erythropoiesis and reduced red cell survival [95].

E/-Osteoporosis

Osteoporosis is a bone disorder characterized by reduced bone strength and bone mineral density (BMD).

Its prevalence in COPD patients is estimated at between 9-75%, depending on the study [96].This prevalence is higher in COPD patients than in a population of healthy subjects or patients with other diseases [97].The majority of studies have revealed a significant inverse relationship between osteoporosis prevalence and FEV1 value [98,99], independently of age, smoking, physical activity and body mass index [100,101].

On the other hand,Ohara et al established a close relationship between the presence of pulmonary emphysema and osteoporosis[102].

The pathogenesis of osteoporosis in COPD, in addition to age, gender and genetic background, is related to the coexistence of several factors such as systemic inflammation, corticosteroid use and vitamin D deficiency [103].

Osteoporotic fractures are common in the elderly, especially in the presence of COPD. They can lead to increased kyphosis and reduced chest wall mobility, promoting deterioration in respiratory function [104].

Osteoporosis associated with COPD leads to significant mortality through fractures and impairs patients' quality of life [104].

F/-Muscular atrophy

Physical inactivity in COPD subjects is the consequence of a sedentary lifestyle that is correlated with muscle dysfunction [105,106].

Reduced physical activity leads to a loss of type I muscle fibers (oxidative, slow and more resistant to fatigue), which defines muscular deconditioning[105].In addition to a sedentary lifestyle, the acquired muscular deterioration of COPD (peripheral myopathy) is linked to oxidative stress[105].

This muscular damage is documented by thigh scans, which show a one-third reduction in cross-sectional area, associated with a halving of quadriceps endurance capacity[106].Muscular atrophy is a predictive factor of mortality in COPD, independent of respiratory function impairment[107] : the 5-year life expectancy of COPD patients with a thigh surface area <70cm2 , at equal FEV1, is 2 times lower, so the prognosis of obstructive disease is linked to quadriceps muscle atrophy.

This structural and functional modification of skeletal muscles impairs activities of daily living and overall quality of life.

G/-Under-nutrition

Undernutrition is common in chronic obstructive pulmonary disease, and is of the proteinocaloric type[108].undernutrition results essentially from resting hypermetabolism, the main cause of which is increased oxygen consumption by the respiratory muscles, the use of medication and the existence of systemic inflammation, whether or not combined with hypoxemia[109].In COPD, undernutrition is directly associated with morbidity (increased frequency of exacerbations)[110] and mortality in

COPD patients, irrespective of respiratory parameters[111,112].The prognostic influence of undernutrition is particularly important in patients with severe obstructive ventilatory disorders, including those with chronic hypoxemia treated with oxygen therapy and/or non-invasive ventilation. The study by Chailleux et al[113], involving over 4,000 patients, showed that a decrease in BMI was associated with an increase in length of stay and risk of hospitalization in patients with chronic respiratory insufficiency receiving home oxygen therapy.

The nutritional status of the COPD patient is assessed by calculating the body mass index (BMI) weight (kg)/m2.BMI is integrated into the BODE index proposed in 2004 to assess the severity of the disease in general [114].It represents a new means of classifying and monitoring the evolution of COPD patients, more relevant than any isolated index for assessing the severity of the disease. Nutritional assessment is therefore essential today, as it helps to define the functional and vital prognosis of patients. However, we know that some patients may be above or below BMI limits and still be in good health, while others may be within these limits and present a nutritional imbalance. Measuring height and weight is not enough. In particular, it is vital to identify sarcopenic obese patients, who are characterized by an excess of body fat associated with a loss of lean body mass. Assessment of the nutritional status of COPD patients should be based on an analysis of body composition (measurement of lean mass and fat mass), which can be carried out using anthropometric measurements (skinfold measurements) [115], DEXA or bioelectrical impedancemetry.

H/-Anxiety disorders and depression.

COPD affects more than just a patient's respiratory function. These repercussions can be observed in the presence of anxiety and depressive disorders at different times in the history of the disease[116], with a prevalence of 50% for anxiety disorders and 33% for depressive disorders[116,117].

Anxiety corresponds to a subjective state of distress, a painful feeling of expectation and apprehension of a danger that is both imminent and imprecise [118].it is reflected in COPD by psychobehavioral changes (agitation, fatigue, irritability, rapid speech, slower concentration and sleep disturbance).

Pathophysiologically, the literature highlights the contribution of pro-inflammatory cytokines (contributing to loss of energy, irritability and feelings of demoralization), emotional dysregulation, increased sympathetic system activity, hypoxia and oxidative stress [119,120,121].

Anxiety and depressive symptoms impair the health-related quality of life of COPD patients[122].these disorders increase the frequency of exacerbations[121] and hospitalizations[122], and prolong the length of hospital stays[123].

In addition, anxiety and depression impair compliance [124], degrade exercise tolerance [235], encourage health-risk behaviour and aggravate feelings of fatigue [125].

Routine clinical assessment of these disorders is becoming essential, particularly to understand the singular and unstable experience of this complex respiratory illness. A reliable and sensitive self-administered questionnaire, the HAD (hospitalization anxiety depression), is available[126].

PART 2: PRACTICAL STUDY

PATIENTS AND METHODS

Introduction

Chronic obstructive pulmonary disease (COPD) is characterized by peripheral flow limitation secondary to smoke or gas inhalation. Its natural history is punctuated by episodes of worsening symptoms known as "exacerbations". Its severity and negative impact are such that it is part of the criteria for defining COPD according to GOLD 2017[122].

However, the definition of an exacerbation remains unambiguous, and the medical community at the Aspen Consensus[122] opted for a clear and pragmatic definition, defining it as an episode of sudden increase in symptoms of dyspnea, cough and/or sputum, lasting more than 24 hours, and requiring modification of the usual treatment.

The occurrence of a COPD exacerbation and the repetition of these episodes are factors with a poor prognosis. Moreover, COPD exacerbations are a source of deterioration in patients' respiratory function and quality of life.

Our aim in this study is to assess the frequency of exacerbations as a function of the stage of severity, to identify the frequent exacerbator profile and to evaluate its impact on the decline in forced expiratory volume in the 1st second (FEV1) and on quality of life.

The secondary objectives are to evaluate the frequency of comorbidities, their distribution according to the severity of the disease and their impact on the quality of life of COPD subjects.

Patients and methods

This is an observational, prospective, epidemiological cohort study involving 135 patients in the Pneumology Department. Patients will be followed for 3 years. Diagnosis of COPD has already been confirmed by spirometry in accordance with GOLD recommendations, and stratification according to COPD severity stage (I, II, III, IV). Follow-up of these patients is based on spirometry performed at least once a year after an exacerbation, a 6-minute walk test and a dyspnea scale score (mMRC). Biological tests are carried out once a year to check for diabetes, anaemia or renal pathology (blood glucose, BH, urea and creatinemia), and to monitor disease progression by measuring CRP.

A quality of life questionnaire (CAT) translated into Arabic is completed by the patient after prior consent.

Inclusion criteria

-COPD subjects with exacerbation criteria as defined (Aspen consensus)

Exclusion criteria

-Acute dyspnea in COPD patients secondary to the occurrence of pneumothorax, pleurisy, infectious pneumonitis or pulmonary embolism, heart failure that may simulate a COPD exacerbation

-Exacerbations due to respiratory pathologies (bronchial dilatation, diffuse interstitial lung disease and bronchial asthma).

Statistical analysis

Data management and statistical analysis will be carried out using SPSS software (version 21). The descriptive analysis of qualitative and ordinal variables will include the number and frequency of each modality with its 95% confidence interval. Quantitative variables will include mean, standard deviation and their confidence intervals, as well as median, percentiles and extreme values. A threshold of 3 exacerbations per year has been proposed to characterize a frequent exacerbator, with reference to the literature [22]. The search for discriminating variables can be carried out using a multivariate logistic regression model, with "frequent exacerbator" as the dependent variable.

Results

For this study, we adopted the Aspen Consensus definition of exacerbation. It is based on respiratory symptoms: dyspnea, cough, sputum. Positive diagnosis was based solely on clinical findings, although additional tests (standard X-ray, D-dimer, cardiac echocardiography) were carried out in certain situations to rule out a differential diagnosis (pneumothorax, pulmonary embolism, heart failure). These confirmed cases were excluded from the study.

Table 5: Characteristics of the study population

	Frequency
Average age (years)	61±9
Male/Female	132/03
Smoking status	
Smoker	66(48.9%)
Ex-smoker	66(48.9%)
No smoking	03(2.2%)
Dyspnea (mMRC)	1.8 ±0.7
Average BMI (kg/m2)	22.1±3.7
Mean FEV1(%)	58.25±15.29
Stage I	7
Stage II	86
Stage III	37
Stage IV	5
Average TM6(m)	366±107
Average BODE index	2.78 ±1
Comorbidity factors	

Values are expressed as mean ± confidence interval

One hundred and thirty-five COPD patients were included: 132 males and 3 females with a mean age of 61 years.49% were ex-smokers and 49% were smokers.COPD subjects varied in severity according to GOLD stage. The mean distance covered during TM6 was 366 m and the mean value of the BODE index was 2.78. Comorbidities were present, with a predominance of cardiovascular diseases (20.7%). The characteristics of the cohort are summarized in table 5.

During our follow-up, we recorded all exacerbations recorded on the department's on-call register and those reported by patients who were managed by peripheral health centers.

The mean frequency of exacerbations was 2.41± 1 exacerbations per year, with a minimum value of 0 and a maximum of 8(fig: 2).

Seventeen percent of COPD patients had no exacerbations and 50.4% were frequent exacerbators (more than 2 exacerbations per year).

Figure 2: Frequency of exacerbations in a series of 135 patients

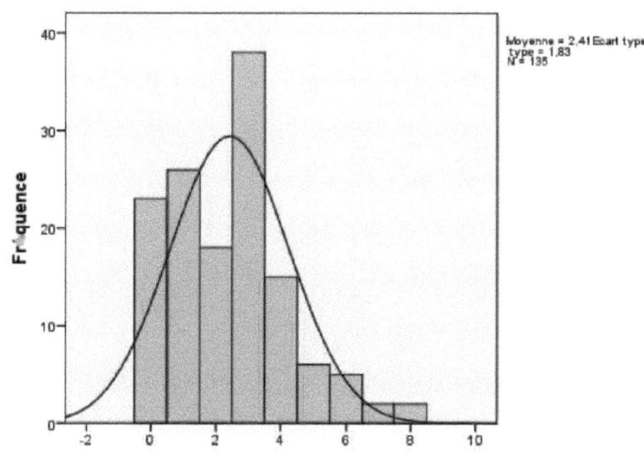

In our study population, we found that COPD sufferers in the severe and very severe stages of the disease had frequent exacerbations (more than 3 per year), compared with COPD sufferers with mild to moderate disease. (The median number of exacerbations increased as the GOLD stages progressed.

Figure 3: The box plots show the distribution of exacerbations according to GOLD stages. The central black lines represent the median.

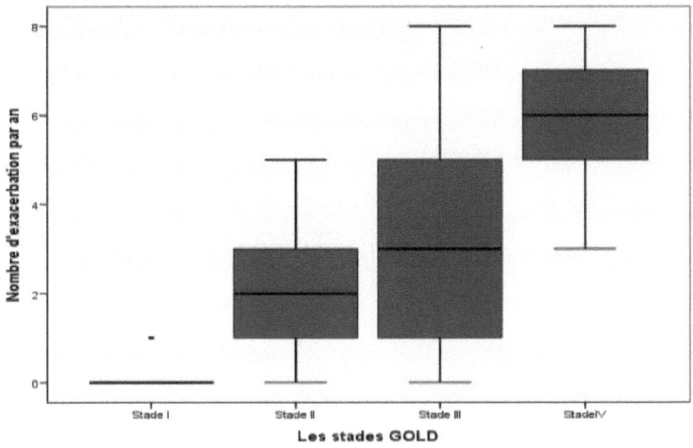

The frequency of exacerbations is highly correlated with severity stage, with a SD p<0.000.More than half of frequent exacerbators are stage III COPD subjects and 100% of stage IV.

Table 6: Distribution of exacerbation frequency by GOLD stage

Average frequency	Stage I (n :7)	Stage II (n :86)	Stage III (n :37)	Stage IV (n :5)
of exacerbations/year	0.14	2.07	3.08	5.80

As the severity of COPD increases, so does the frequency of exacerbations (table 6).

To determine the impact of these acute episodes on lung function, we assessed the annual decline in forced expiratory volume in the first second (FEV1) in COPD patients in two categories: frequent exacerbators $\geq 3EX^n$ and those with fewer exacerbations < 3EX /year.

Table 7: Average decline in FEV1 according to frequency of exacerbations

	Frequency of exacerbations	Decline medium FEV1	T	P	P<0.05	95% CI
	<3EX/AN	34.22 ±24				
	≥ 3EX/AN	44.41 ± 20				
COPD			-2.61	0.008	**	[-17.8,-2]

Shown are the correlation coefficients (= t)** p < 0.005; significant -IC 95%: confidence interval.FEV1:forced expiratory volume in the 1st second.EX: Exacerbations

T-test analysis of the data shows that the decline in FEV1 in frequent exacerbators is 44.41ml, higher than that in COPD patients with fewer exacerbations 34.22ml. The difference between these two categories of COPD is highly significant(T:-2.61, P <0.05)(Table:3).

Figure 4 shows that there is no overlap between the confidence interval of mean FEV1 decline in COPD subjects with frequent exacerbations (≥ 3EX/year) and those with fewer exacerbations (<3 ex/year).

Figure 4: Error bars for mean FEV1 decline and frequency of exacerbations

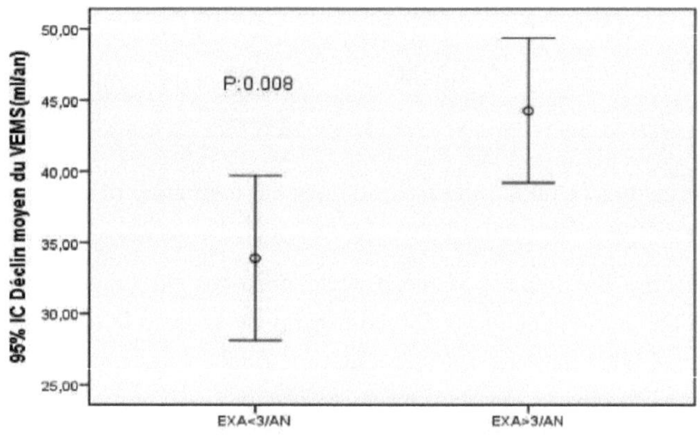

The quality of life of COPD patients is assessed by the sore CAT. This questionnaire includes various items on cough, expectoration, dyspnoea and sleep quality. Our survey shows that the score varies from 7 to 37, with an

average of 16.42 ± 6.67, indicating that the quality of life of our COPD patients is impaired on average (fig. 5).

CAT scores were compared between the two populations of frequent and less frequent exacerbators.

Figure 5: CAT score frequency in a series of 135 COPD patients

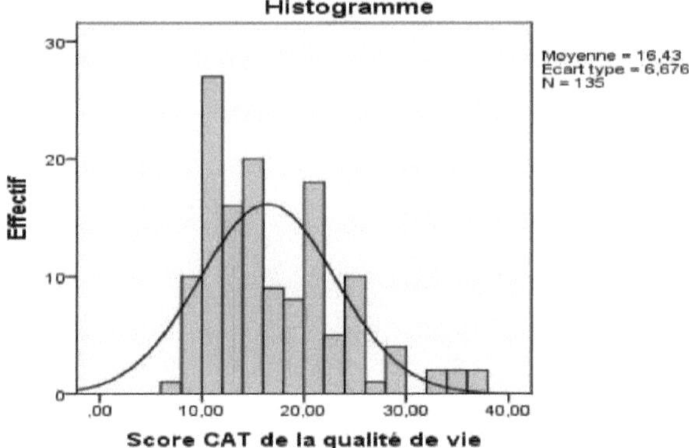

Figure 6: Boxplots showing the distribution of the CAT score according to the frequency of exacerbations.

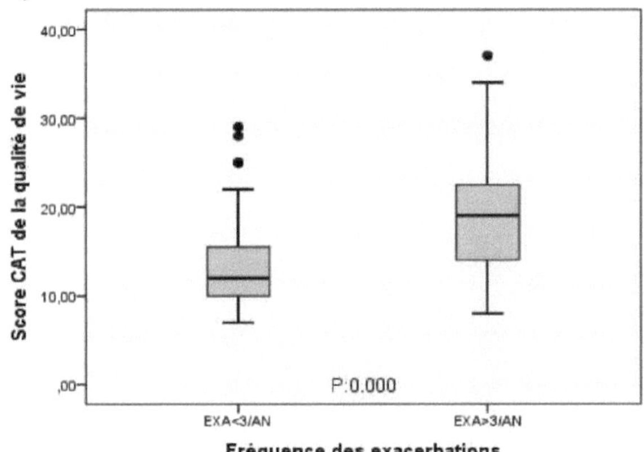

These results show that recurrent exacerbations in COPD patients make a major contribution to their reduced quality of life.

Comorbidity factors

During the follow-up period, 63 cases of extra-respiratory manifestations were identified. Cardiovascular factors represent the most frequent systemic manifestation, followed by diabetes (Fig: 7).

Figure 7: Distribution of comorbidities in COPD patients

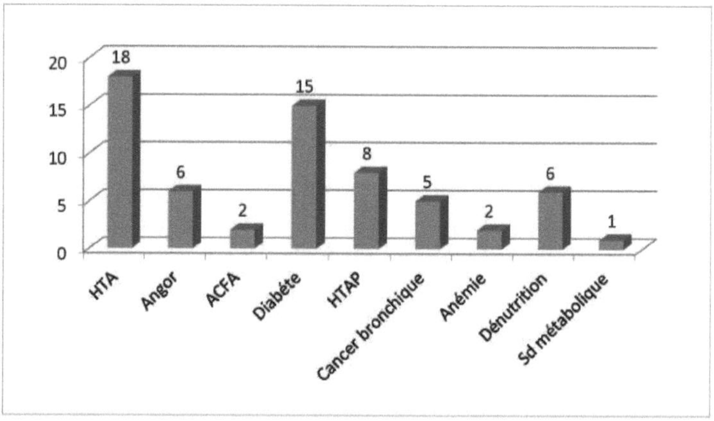

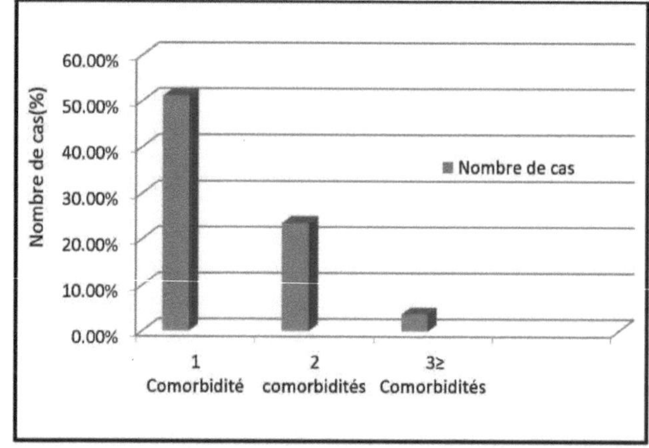

The frequency of comorbidities in COPD subjects is divided into 39% of cases with a single comorbidity, 16% of cases with 2 comorbidities and 3.7% of cases with more than 2 comorbidities (Fig: 8).

Figure 8: Distribution of COPD subjects according to the frequency of comorbidities

Comorbidity factors and severity stages (GOLD)

According to the results of our study, the frequency of comorbidities in COPD patients increases with the severity of the disease; it is more frequent in stages III and IV, with rates of 70.3% and 80% respectively (fig. 9).

Figure 9: Distribution of comorbidities by severity stage (GOLD)

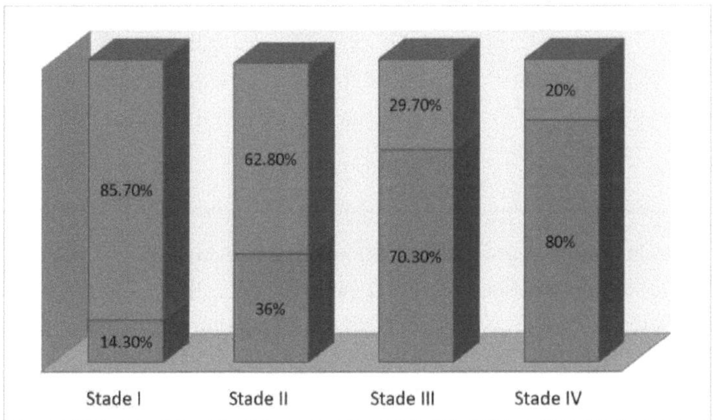

Based on comparison with the Pearson test, there is a significant correlation between the frequency of comorbidities and COPD severity stages (DS ,P :0.001).The more advanced the disease stage, the greater the frequency of comorbidities in COPD patients.

Quality of life and co-morbidities

According to the cross-tabulation between CAT sore and the presence or absence of associated pathologies, a higher score is observed in half of COPD patients with comorbidities, and a lower score in 31.5% of COPD patients without comorbidities.

These results show that quality of life as assessed by the CAT score is impaired in COPD patients with comorbidities compared to those without systemic manifestations (fig: 10).

Figure 10: CAT score distribution according to the presence or absence of comorbidities

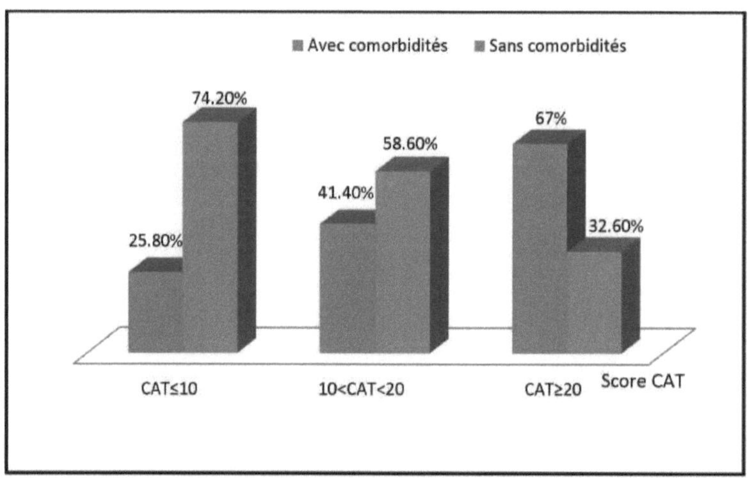

There was a highly significant relationship between CAT score and the presence of comorbidities in COPD patients (P : 000). The presence of cormobidities in COPD patients contributes to an altered quality of life

CAT score by frequency of comorbidities

We wanted to know the impact of the frequency of comorbidities on the quality of life of COPD subjects, so we divided COPD patients into 3 groups according to the number of extra-respiratory manifestations present per patient.

Figure 11 shows that the CAT score increases as the number of associated pathologies increases, with a high score for patients with 3 comorbidities in 100% of cases and a lower score for those with only one or two.

The relationship between the frequency of co-morbidities and quality of life is highly correlated (p<0.05), which means that the more COPD sufferers suffer from several illnesses, the more their quality of life is impaired.

Figure 11: CAT score by number of comorbidities

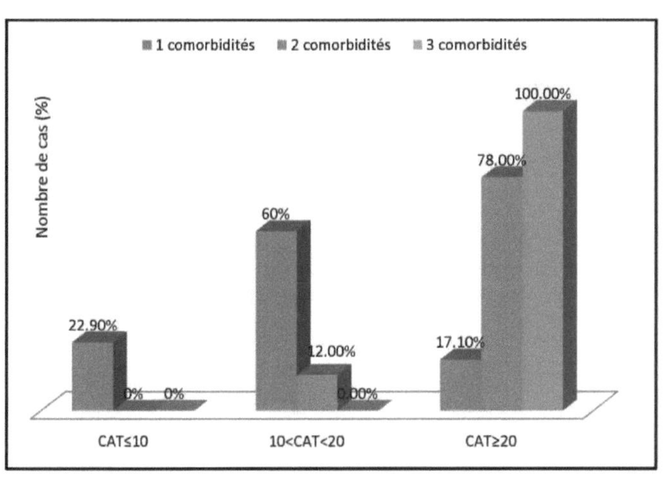

1 comorbidités
2 comorbidités
3 comorbidités
Nombre de cas (%)
22,90%
0%
0%
60%
12.00%
0.00%
17.10%
78.00%
100.00%
CAT≤10
10<CAT<20
CAT≥20

Discussion

The frequency of exacerbations varies according to the definition used, with an incidence twice as high if the symptom-based definition is used rather than the operational definition based on the use of systemic corticosteroid and/or antibiotic therapy. They are frequent, costly and a source of morbidity and mortality. What's more, they have been associated with a more rapid decline in respiratory function and quality of life, and even with excess long-term mortality. The main etiologies of exacerbations are tracheobronchial infections, more viral than bacterial, which explains the frequency of exacerbations during the peak of viral epidemics between November and February. However, the absence of an identifiable cause is frequent in a third of cases.

During the study period, 322 exacerbations were recorded, with an average rate of 2.4±2 exacerbations per year. Twenty-three patients (17%) had no exacerbations during follow-up. Our results are similar to the literature, which reports a median exacerbation rate of 2.5-3 per year [27,38].

COPD exacerbations are recurrent events occurring at any stage of the disease, but according to the literature, their frequency and severity increase with disease severity [26,28,29]. This is in line with our findings of a close correlation between severity stage and frequency of exacerbations (P<0.05), with the mean annual rate of exacerbations increasing with disease severity, the mean rate for stage III being 3.08 higher than that for stage II 2.07.

All these data concur with the work of Donaldson et al [26] with a follow-up of two and a half years, showed that the annual rate of exacerbations in severe COPD was higher than those with moderate to severe COPD with respective values of 2.7 and 3.4.

The association between the frequency of exacerbations and the severity of COPD is probably linked to a permanent bacterial colonization favored by severe bronchial obstruction, which maintains this condition in a vicious circle, with each exacerbation leading to another.

Since FEV(L) is the gold standard for monitoring the evolution of lung function, all our COPD subjects underwent spirometry at least once a year in the stable state.

According to our functional results,the decline in FEV1 is more marked in frequent exacerbators, with a difference of 10ml compared with less frequent exacerbators.the same results have been obtained in other studies[29].a greater decline25ml versus 46ml was found in a prospective trial [26] including 109 COPD patients followed for 04 years.

Conversely, a weaker effect was obtained in the ECLIPSE study [122], with a fall in FEV1 of 2 ± 0.5 ml per year.

However, other studies have not shown any impact on lung function, as the population studied is essentially composed of mild-to-moderate stages, in whom exacerbations are less frequent. [123]

From a pathophysiological standpoint, exacerbations are an enhancement of the pre-existing airway inflammation that is at the root of bronchospasm. These inflammatory processes, which recur over time, aggravate bronchospasm and accelerate the decline in FEV1.

Parker et al [35] demonstrated that increased distension predominated in the assessment of 20 COPD patients after a moderate exacerbation. In our work, measurements of thoracic distension were not explored.

The CAT questionnaire was translated into dialectal Arabic to ensure that it could be easily understood by patients, who gave their prior consent to take part in the questionnaire. For subjects with a low level of education, the questionnaire was completed by the doctor in collaboration with the patient.

Given that our population is made up mainly of patients with moderate to severe COPD, the mean CAT score is high (16.42), suggesting that our patients' quality of life is already impaired at a moderate stage of the disease. Our results are similar to those of a study using the same quality-of-life assessment tool, carried out in 400 COPD subjects of all stages [124].

The present study demonstrated a very close correlation between the frequency of exacerbations and quality of life (r: 0.46, p<0.01), as prolonged persistence of dyspnea and cough significantly reduces daily activity and impairs sleep quality. Symptoms of exacerbation regress very slowly, even weeks to a month after the episode. The consequences are even more serious in the case of recurrent exacerbations, where quality of life scores do not improve rapidly, as Spencer et al[125] showed in a prospective 6-month study that quality of life scores, as assessed by the Saint Georges questionnaire, only recovered gradually over 6 months.Similarly, when another exacerbation occurred, these scores corrected only very slowly, with the result that at 6 months, these patients had still not recovered their baseline values, unlike patients who had only had one exacerbation.

Over a 3-year follow-up period, we identified 63 cases of comorbidities (46%5), some of which were discovered during exacerbations and others during routine annual check-ups. The most frequent extra-respiratory manifestations were cardiovascular factors (41%) (arterial hypertension, angina, ACFA).

The prevalence of co-morbidities is very high, at 63-85% [6].according to the literature, COPD patients are at high risk of cardiovascular disease, the most frequent being hypertension, heart failure, coronary heart disease and vascular accidents[66,81].these are among the main causes of death in COPD subjects.

The present study showed a significant relationship between disease severity stages and the frequency of comorbidities (P<0.05), the latter increasing with the severity of bronchial obstruction. Our results are consistent with those found by the Rw.Dalnegro team [126].

To highlight the impact of comorbidities on the quality of life of COPD subjects, the CAT score was assessed, and was higher in subjects with extrapulmonary manifestations.There is a highly significant correlation between quality of life and comorbidities. There seems to be an additive effect of quality of life impairment in the presence of several pathologies associated with COPD.

Conclusion

Exacerbations weigh heavily on the progression of the disease: they accelerate the decline in lung function and contribute to a deterioration in quality of life.

Preventing exacerbations is a major objective of COPD treatment, and one which we hope will have a beneficial influence on the natural history of the disease. It is essential to reduce the frequency and severity of these episodes through smoking cessation and influenza and pneumococcal vaccination.

On the other hand, as is classically accepted, COPD is accompanied by extra-respiratory manifestations, with cardiovascular pathologies dominating and grafting the vital prognosis of COPD patients.The systematic search for associated pathologies is necessary in our daily practice of managing patients suffering from COPD.

It is a disabling pathology marked by profound impairment of daily quality of life at all stages of severity, with various components: dyspnea, fatigue, anxiety, depression and cognitive disorders. This fact justifies a palliative approach for elderly COPD sufferers in the same way as for cancer patients.

References

1- N.Roche,G.Huchon.Epidemiology of chronic bronchopneumopathy obstructive.Rev Prat(13)2004,1408-1413.

2- A. Lopez, C. C. Murray. 1998. The global burden of disease, 1990-2020. *Nat.Med.* 4:1241-1243.

3- C.Fuhrman ,MC. Delmas. Descriptive epidemiology of chronic obstructive pulmonary disease (COPD) in France. Revue des Maladies Respiratoires

4 -T Similowski et al.Press Med 2003

5- R.Kessler ,E.Weitznblum.BPCO :Les premiers symptômes à l'insuffisance respiratoire chronique.Rev Prat2004 ;13 ;1414-1417

6- G.Fumagalli,F.Fabiani,S.Fortet al.INDACO Projet.COPD and link between comorbidities,lung function and inhalation therapy Multidisciplinary Respiratory Med 2015,19;4

7- AG. Wheaton,ES.Ford,TJ.Cunningham,JB.Croft .COPD,hospital visits and comorbidities national survey of residential care facilities 2010.J Aging Health 2015,27:480-99

8- E.Marchand,G.Maury.Evaluation of COPD Assessment CAT in COPD patients.Rev Mal Respir 2012(29) ;391-397

9- T.Perez,P.Serrier,C.Prisk, A.Mahdad.COPD and quality of life.Rev Mal Respir 2013(30),22-32

10- American Thoracic Society / European Respiratory Society Task Force.Standards for the Diagnosis and Management of Patients with COPD [Internet] Version 1.2. American Thoracic Society. Am J Respir Crit Care Med 1995 ;152 :s77-s21.

1 1. R A.Pauwels,A. S. Buist, P. M. Calverley, C. R. Jenkins, S. S. Hurd, and GOLD Scientific Committee. 2001. Global Strategy for the Diagnosis, Management, and Prevention of Chronic Obstructive Pulmonary Disease . NHLBI/WHO GlobalInitiative for Chronic Obstructive Lung Disease (GOLD) Workshop Summary. *Am.J.Respir.Crit.Care Med.* 163:1256-1276.

12- KF.Rabe,S.Hurd, A Anzueto et al.Global Strategy for the diagnosis,management and prevention of COPD.GOLD excutive summary Am J Respir Crit Care Med 2007,176 ;532-55

13- Global initiative for chronic obstructive lung disease.Gloabal initiative for COPD:a global strategy for the diagnosis,management and prevention of COPD 2016.

14- SPLF.Definition,classification,prognostic factors. Rev Mal Respir(2010),27,S11-S18.

15- PR.Burgel,P.Nesme-Meyer,P.Chanez,D.Caillaud,P.Carre,T.Perez et al.Cough and sputum production are associated with frequent exacerbations and hos^pitalizations in COPD subjects.Chest 2009,135 :975-82.

16- J.Vestbo,P.Lange.Can GOLD stage 0 provide information of prognostic value in COPD ?Am J Respir Crit Care Med 2002 ;166 :329-32.

17- M.Fournier.Emphysema.Rev Prat (13)2004 ;1419-1423.

18- L.Joos,PD.Paré, AJ. Sandford.Genetic risk factors of COPD. Swiss Med Wkly 2002:132:27-37

19- A.Cuvelier,D.Benhamou,b. Lamia ,JF.Muir.Exacerbations of COPD EMC

20- TA. Seemungal, GC.Donaldson, A.Bhowmik Et al.Time course and recovery of exacerbations in patients with COPD.Am J Respir Crit Care Med 2000 ;161 :1608-13

21- C.Fletcher,R. Peto: The natural history of chronic airflow obstruction. *BMJ* 1977; 1: 1645-8.

22- CG.Donaldson,TA. Seemungal, A.Bhowmik et al.Relationship between exacerbation frequency and lung function decline in COPD.Thorax 2002,57 ;847-52

23- RE.Kanner,NR.Anthonisen,JE.Connett et al.Lower respiratory illnesses promote FEV(1) decline in current smokers but not ex-smokers with mild COPD ;Results from the lung health study.Am J Respir Crit Care Med 2001 ;164 :358-64.

24- R.Rodriguez-Roisin Toward a consensus definition for COPDexacerbations Chest 2000,117 ;3985-4015.

25- PW.Jones ,WH.Chen, et al.Characterising and quantifying the symptomatic features of COPD exacerbations.Chest 2011 ;139 :1388-94

26- GC.Donaldson,JA. Wedzicha. COPD exacerbations: Epidemiology. Thorax 2006;61:164-8

27- E.Sapey,RA. Stockley. COPD exacerbations2: Aetiology. Thorax 2006;61:250-8.

28- R.Kessler,A.Chaouat,AS.Bugnet,M.Canuet,E.Weitzenblum Exacerbations. Initial evaluation. In: Huchon G, Roche N, editors.Broncho-pneumopathies chroniques obstruc-tives. Paris: Margaux Orange; 2003p. 669-81

29- PW.JOnes,LR. Willits ,PS.Burge ,PM. Calverley,on behalf of the inhaled steroids in ob-structive lung disease in Europe studyinvestigators. Disease severity and the effect offluticasone propionate on chronic obstruc-tive pulmonary disease exacerbations. Eur RespirJ2003;21:68-73.

30- Ministère de la Santé et des Solidarités.Programme d'actions en faveur de la broncho-pneumopathie chronique obstruc-tive (BPCO), 2005- 2010,(Connaitre,prévenie et mieux prendre en charge la BPCO "15novembre 200

31- T.Similowski,N.Roche. Practical management of patients with COPD. COPD: definition and impact. Paris: JohnLibbey Eurotext; 2006.

32- DE.Hilleman,N.Dewan et al.Pharmacoeconomic evaluation of COPD Chest 2000118 ;1278-85

33- F.Anderson,S.Borg et al.The costs of exacerbations in COPDRespir Med 2002 ;96 ;700-8

34- J.Haughney,MR.Partridge et al.Exacerbations of COPD quantifying the patients' perspective using discrete choice modelling.Eur Respir J 2005 ;26 :623-9

3 5-CM.Parker,N. Voduc, SD. Aaron et al.Physiological changes during symptom recovery from moderate exacerbations of COPD.Eur Respir J 2005 ;26 :420-8

36- NJ.Stevenson,PP.Walker,RW.Costello et al.Lung mechanics and dyspnea during exacerbations of COPD.Am J Respir Crit Care Med 2005 ;172 ;1510-

37- MK.Johnson,M.Birch,R.Carter et al.Measurement of physiological recovery from exacerbations of COPD using within-breath forced oscillometry.Thorax 2007,62 ;299-32.

38- Société de Pneumologie de Langue Française. Recommendations for the management of obstructive pulmonary disease. Rev Mal Respir. 2003;20:294-329.

39- CG.Cote,LJ.Dordelly,BR.Celli .Impact of COPD exacerbations on patients centered outcomes.Chest 2007 :131 :696-704.

40- CG.Cote,VM.Pinto-Plata,JM.Marin.The modufied BODE index :validation with mortality in COPD.Eur Respir J 2008 ;32 :1269-74

41- N.Roche,B.Aguilaniu,PR.Burgel et al.Prevention of COPD exacerbations:a fundamental issue.Rev Mal Respir 2012,29 ;756-774.

42- JR.Feary,LC.Rodrigues,CJ. Smith et al.Prevalence of major comorbidities in subjects with COPD and incidence of myocardial infarction and stoke ;a comprehensive analysis using data from primary care .Thorax 2010 ;65 :956-62

43- GC.Donaldson, JR.Hurst, CJ. Smith et al .Increased risk of myocardial infarction and stroke following exacerbation of COPD.Chest 2010 ;137 :1091-7

44- CR.Meier ,SS.Jick,LE.Derby et al.Acute respiratory infections and risk of first time acute myocardial infaction.Lancet 1998 ;351 :1467-71

45- TC.Clayton,M.Thompson,W.Meade.Recent respiratory infection and risk of cardiovascular disease :case control study through a general practice database.Eur Heart J 2008,29 ;96-103.

46-   L.HuiartL,P.Ernest,X.Ranouil et al.Oral corticosteroid use and the risk of acute myocardial infarction in COPD.Can Respir J 2006 ;13 ;134-8

47-   NM.Hawkins,D.Wang,MC. Petrie et al.CHARM investigators and Commettees.Baseline characteristics and outcomes of patients with heart failure receiving bronchodilators in the CHARM programme.Eur JHeart Fail 2010,12 :557- 65.

48-   S.Salpeter,TM.Ormiston,E.Salpeter et al.Cardioselective betablokers for COPD.Cochrane Database sust Rev 20054 :CD003566.

49-   CL.Chang,SC.Robinson, GD.Mills et al.Biochemical markers of cardiac dysfunction predict mortality in acute exacerbations of COPD.Thorax 2011 ;66 ;764- 8.

50-   J.Bourbeau,G.Ford,H.Zackon et al.Impact of patients health status following early identification of COPD exacerbations.Eur Respir J 2007 ;30 ;907-13

51-   S.Spencer,PM.Calverly,PS.Burger et al.Impact of preventing exacerbations on deterioration of health status in COPD Eur Respir J2004,23 :698-702

52-   S.De Miranda,F.Pochard,M. Chaize et al.Postinintensive care unit psychological burden in patients with COPD and informal caregivers ;a multicenter study.Crit Care Med 2011 ;39 :112-8

53-   A.Rabbat ,A.Guetta et al.Management of acute COPD exacerbations.Rev Mal Respir 2010 ;10 :939-59

54-   DM.Manninno,DE.Doherty, S.Buist A. Global Initiative onobstructive Lung Disease(GOLD) classification of lung disease and mortality ;findings from the atherosclerosis risk in communities(ARIC) study.Respir Med 2006 ;100 :115-22

55-   M.Hoogendoom,RT.Hoogendoom et al.Case fatality of COPD exacerbations, a meta-analysis and statitiscal modelling approach.Eur Respir J 2011 ;37 ;508-15

56- National Collaborating Centre for Chronic Conditions Chronic obstructive pulmonary disease. National clinical guideline on management of chronic obstructive pulmonary disease in adults in primary and secondary care *Thorax* 2004; 59: 1232206

57-   AR.Falsey,PA.Hennessey et al.Respiratory syncitial virus infection in elderly and high-risk adults.N Engl J Med 2005 ;352 :1749-59.

58-   C.Beadling,MK.Slifka et al.How do viral infectuons predispose patients to bacterial infections?Curr Opin Infec Dis 2004 ;17 :185-91

59-   LM.Fabbri,KF.Rabe.From COPD to chronic systemic imflammatory syndrome?Lancet 2007;370:797-9.

60-   M.Charlson,RE.Charlson,W.Briggs,J.Hollenberg:Can disease management target patients most likely to generate high costs?The impact of comorbidity. J. Gen Interm Med 2007;22:464-9.

61- PR.Burgel.Role of comorbidities in the evolution of COPD.Rev Mal Respir 2008,25;11-15

62- DD.Sin,L.Wu,SF.Man;The realation ship between reduced lung faction and cardiovascular mortality;a population-based study and a systemic review of the literature.Chest 2005;127:1952-9.

63- AG.Agusti.Systemic effects of COPD.Proc Am.Thorax Soc 2005;2;367-706

64- Global Inititive for the diagnosis,management and prevention of chronic obstructive pulmonary disease.htpp://www.goldcopd.com/Guidelineitem.asp.

65- PMA.Calverley,JA.Anderson,B.Celli,GT.Ferguson,C.Jenkins,PW.Jones,and al.Cardiovascular events in patients with COPD:TORCH Study results.Thorax 2010;65:719-25.

66- DM.Mannino,D.Thorn,A.Swensen,F.Holguin.Prevalence and outcomes of dibetes,hypertention and cardiovascular disease in COPD.Eur Respir J 2008.32/962-9

67- A.Corlateanu,J.Kocks,T.Van Der Molen, V.Botnaru. Comorbidities and disease specific health status in young and old COPD patients.Eur Respir Congress 2009(abstract E503).

68- PR.Burgel,JL.Paillasseur,D.Caillaud,I.Tillie-Leblond,P.Chanez,R.Escamilla,et al.Clinical COPD phenotypes; a novel approach using principal component and cluster analyses.Eur REespir J 2010;36:531-9

69- Di Francia M,Barbier D et al.Tumor necrosis factor alpha levels and weight loss in COPD.Am J Respir Crit Care Med 1994;150;1453-5

70- CG.Donaldson,TA.Seemungal,IS.Patel et al. AAirway and systemic inflammation and decline in lung function in patients with COPD.Chest 2005;128;1995-2004.

70-DD.Sin ,R.Leung et al.Circulatting surfactant protein D as a potential lung specific boimaker of heath outcomes in COPD:a pilot study .BMC Pulm Med 2007;7:13

71- S.Bozinovski,A.Hutchinson et al.Serum amyloid is a biomarker of acute exacerbations of COPD.Am J Respir Crit Care Med 2008;177;269-78

72- G.Prevot,G.Plat ,J.Maziers.COPD and bronchial cancer.Epidemiological and biological links.Rev Mal Respir 2012(29);545-556.

73- A.Couillard,D.Veale,J-F.Muir.Comorbidities in COPD ;Anew challenge in clinical practice.Rev Pneumol Clin 2011,67 ;143-153.

74- M. Yanai, J.Hatazawa,F. Ojima, et al.Deposition and clearance of inhaled 18FDG powder in patients with COPD.Eur Respir J 1998;11;1342-1348.

75- SS.Islam,D. Schotten feld.Declining FEV1 and chronic productive cough in cigarette smokers.A 25-year prospective study of lung cancer, incidence inTecumsch Michigan.Cancer Epidemiol Biomarkers Prev 1994;3:289-298.

76- DM.Manino,SW.Aguayo,TL.Petty,SC.Redd.Low lung function and incident lung cancer in the united states data-from the first National Health and Nutrition Examination Survey follow-up.Arch Inter Med 20008,163:1475-80.

77- S.wasswa-Kintu,WQ.Gan,SF.Man,PD.Pare,DD.Sin.Relatioship between reduced forced expiratory volume in one second and the risk of lung cancer;a systematic review and meta-analysis.Thorax 2005,60;570-5.

78- DO.Wilson,JL.Weissfeld,A.Balkan,et al. association of radiographic emphysema and airflow obstruction with lung cancer.AM J Respir Crit Care Med 2008;178:738- 744.

79- KG.Alberti,PZ.Zimmet.For the WHO consultation.Definition,diagnosis and classification od diabetes mellitus and its complications.PartI.Diagnosis and classification of diabetes mellitus.Provisional Report of WHO consultation.Diabet Med 1998,15:539-53

80- JS.Rana,MA.Mittleman,J.Sheik,FB.Hu,JE.Manson,GA Colditz et al .Copd,asthma and risk of type 2 diabetis in women Diabetis Care 2004,27;247-84.

81- LM.Fabbri,F.Luppi,B.Beghé,KF.Rabe.Complex chronic comorbidities of COPD.Eur Respir J 2008;31:204-12.

82- K.Marquis,F.Maltais,V.Dugua,AM.Bezean,P.LeblancJJobin et al.The metabolic syndrome in patients with COPD.J.Cardio Pulm Rhehabil 2005;25:226-32.

83- J. Spranger, A.Kroke,M.Mohlig,K.Hoffman,MM.Bergmann.M.Risto et al.Results of the prospective population based Europeen Prospective investigation into cancer and Nutrition(EPIC) Protsdam study.Diabetis 2003;52:812-7.

84- H.Watz,B. Waschki, A.Kirsten,KC.Muller, G.Kretschman,T.Meyer et al.The metabolic syndrome in patients with C OPD. Frequency and associated consequences for systemic inflammation and physical inactivity.Chest 2009;136:1039-46.

8 5ES.Ford,MB.Schulz,T.Pischom,MM.Bergmann,HG.Joost,H.Bocing.Metabolic syndrome and risk of incident diabetis: Finding from the European into Cancer and Nutrition-Postsdam study.Cardiovascular diabetol 2008;12-35

86- A.Chambellan,E.Chailleux,T. Similowski.Prognostic value of the hematocrit inchronic respiratory insufficiency. A 20-year analysis of the ANTADIR observatory.Eur Respir Congress 20006A494.

87- C.Cote,MD.Zibliberbrg,SH.Mody,et al.Haemoglobin level and its clinical impact in a cohort of patients with COPD.Eur Respir J 2007;29:923-929.

88- M.John,S.Hoernig,W.Doehmer,et al.Anemia and inflammation in COPDChest

2005;127:825-829

89- A.Chabellan,E.Chailleux,T.Similowski.Prognostic value of the hematocrit in patients with severe COPD receiving long-term oxygen therapy .Chest 2005:128:1201-1208.

9 0DM.Mannino,AF.Shorr,JJDoyle,LS.Stem,LR.Mdoigitser,M.Stergartel,MD Zibiberbeg.Prevalence of anemia in subjects with COPD.Prosc Am Thorac Soc 2006;3:A615.

91- T.Similowski,A.Agust,W MacNce,et al .Potential means impact of anemia of COPD.EUR Respir J 2006.27:390-396.

92- L.Graat-Verboon,EF Wouters,FW Smeenk,BE.Vandenborn,R.Lunde,MA ?Spruit.Current status of search on osteoporosis in COPD Asystematic review.Eur Respir J 2009.34/209-18.

93- A.Vrieze,MH.Degreef,PJ.Wijkstra,JB.Wempe.Low bonemineral density in COPD patients related to worse lung function, low weight and decreased fat-free mass.aOsteoporosis Int 2007,18:1197-202.

94- G. Thabut, G.Dauriat,JB Stern,D.Logeart,A.Levy,R.Marrash-Chahla ,et al Pulmonary hemodynamics in advanced COPD candidates for lung volume reduction in surdery or lung transplantation Chest 2009;127:1531-6.

9 5R. Thurnheer, J.Muntwyler,U.Stammberger,KE.Bloch, A.Zollinger,W. Wederel ,et alCoronary artery disease in patients undergoing lung volume reduction surgery for emphysema Chest 1997;112:122-8.

96- DD.Sin,JP.Man SF.Man.The risk of osteoporosis in Caucasian men and females with COPD.AmJ Med 2003;114:10-4.

97- T.Ohara,T.Hirai,S.Muro,et al .Retionship between pulmonary emphysema and osteoporosis assessed by CT in patients with COPD.Chest 2008;134:1244-9.

98- A.Lehouck,H.Van Remoortel,T.Troosters,M.Decramer,W. Janssens.COPD and metabolism osseus.une mise à jour Clinique .Rev Mal Respir 2010;27:1231-1242.

99- JD. Corter, S.Patel,FL. Sultan,Z J Thompson,H.Margaux, A. Sterret, et al.The recognition and treatment of vertebral fractures in males with COPD.Respir Med 2008 ;102 :1165-72.

1 00- P.Haeritjens,J.Magiaziner,C.S.ColonEmeric,D.Vandersehueren,K.Milisen,B.Velkenin s,et al.Meta-analysis;excess mortality after hip fracture among older women and men.Ann Intern Med 2010;152:380-90.

100- A.Couillard,C.Préfaut.From muscle disude to myopathy in COPD:pototiel contribution of oxidative stress.Eur Respir J2005;26:703.

101- I. Serres, V.Gautier,A.Varray,C. Préfaut. Impaired skeletal muscle endurance related to physical inactivity and altered lung function in COPD patients.Chest 1998 ;113-900.

102- K.Marquis,J.Jobin,F.Maltais,et al.Mid thigh muscle cross-sectional area is a better predictor of mortality than body mass index in patients with COPD.Am J Resir Crit Care Med 2002;166:809.

103- JP.Laabon.Nutrition and COPD.EMC pneumology

104- R.Hallin,LI.Koivisto-hurti,E.Lindberg, et al.Nutritional status dietary energy intake and the risk of exacerbations in patients with COPD.Respir Med 2006,100(3),561-567.

105- R.Hallin,G.Gudmundsson,C.Usuppli et al.Nutritional status and long term mortality in hospitalized patients with COPD.Respir.Med 2007;101(9):1954-1960.

106- EM.Pouw,GP.Tenvelde,BH.Croonem et al.Early non elective readmission for COPD in associated with weight loss.Clin Nutr 2000;19:95-9.

107- E.Chailleux,JP.Laban,D.Veale.Prognostic value of nutritional depletion in patients with COPD treated by long-term oxygen therapy;data from the ANTADIR observatory.Chest 2003;123:1460-6

108- JM.Cano,H.Roth,I.Court-Fortune et al.Clinical research Group of societé francophone de nutrition enterale et parenterale.Nutritional depletion in patients with long term oxygene therapy an/or home mechanical ventilation.Eur Respir J 2002;20:30-3.

109- R. Thibault,E.Legallic,M.Picard-Kossovsky,D.Darman et al. Assessment of nutritional status and body composition in patients with COPD.Comparison of several mrthods.Rev Mal Respir 2010;27(7):693-702.

110- G.Ninot.Anxiety and depression associated with COPD;an issue review.Rev Mal Respir 2010(6):739-748.

111- J.Maurer,V.Rebba pragada, S. Bordon et al. Anxiety and depression in COPD:Current understanding unanswered questions and research needs .Chest 2008,134:43s-56s.

112- KM.Hynninem,MH.Breitve,AB.Wiborg,et al.Psychological characteristics of patients with COPD.A review J.Psychosom Res 2005,59:429-443.

113- CG.Ferguson,M. Stanley,, J. Souchek et al.The utility of somatic symptoms as indicators of depression and anxiety in military veterans with COPD.Depress Anxiety 2006,23:42-49.

114- D.De Ridder,R.Geenen,R.Kujer et al.Psychological adjustment to chronic disease.Lancet 2008,372:246-255.

115- TM.Eagan,T.Ueland,PD.Wagner et al.Systemic inflammatory markers in COPD.Results from the Bergen COPD.Cohort Study .Eur Respir J 2010,35:540-548.

116- K.Hill,R.Gerst,RS.Goldstein et al.Anxiety and depression in end stage COPD.Eur Respir J 2008;31:667-677.

117- E.Breslin,C.Van der Schans,S.breukink et al.Perception of fatigue and quality of life in patients with COPD.Chest 1998;114:958-964.

118- P.Almagro,B.Barreira,A?Ochoa de Echagrein.Risk factors for hospital readmission in patients with COPD.Respiration 2006,73:311-317.

119- W.X,J.Collet,S.Shapiro et al.India.pendant effect of depression and anxiety on COPD exacerbations and hospital.AM J Respir Crit Care Med 2008,178:913-920.

120- I.Bjellanda,A.Dahlb,T.TangenHangc et al.The validity of the hospital anxiety and depression scale.An updated literature Review J Psychosom Res 2002;52:69-77

121- J.Vestbo,LD.Edwards,PD.Scanlon et al.Changes in forced expiratory volume in 1 second over time in COPD.N Engl J Med 2011,365(13),1184-1192.

122- M.Nishimura,H.Makita,K.Nagai et al .Annual change in pulmonary function and clinical phenotype in COPD.Am J Respir Crit Care Med 2012(185(1);44-52.

123- JP.De Torres,C.Casanova,C.Hernandez et al.Gender associated differences in determinants of quality of life in patients with COPD.A case series study health qual Life Outcomes 2006,4;72

124- Oussedik.F et al.The impact of exacerbations on respiratory function.Rev Mal Respir jan 2016(33).183-184

125- Dal Negro RW, Bonadiman L, Turco P. Prevalence of different comorbidities in COPD patients by gender and GOLD stage. *Multidiscip Respir Med.* 2015 Aug 5;10(1):24.

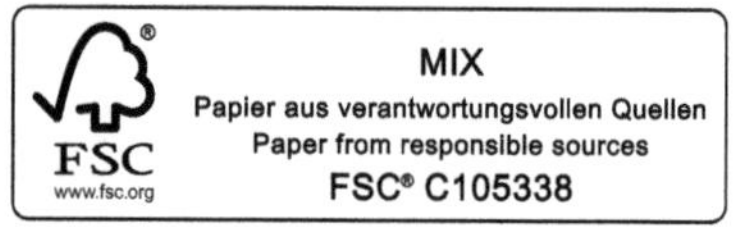

Printed by Books on Demand GmbH, Norderstedt / Germany